DAILY VAGUS NERVE EXERCISES

JAI CYR

Table of Contents

CHAPTER 6
EXERCISES

BONUS EXERCISES
MUSCLE RELAXATION TECHNIQUES

ACCESS YOUR EXERCISE DEMONSTRATION AND
INSTRUCTION VIDEO WITH THIS QR CODE

"It doesn't matter how much you drive around, you will never get to where you want to go if you don't have the right map."

STANLEY ROSENBERG

Chapter 1
Introduction

If you are like me and most people out there, you would like to live a happier and easier life. A life that feels more peaceful, joyful, and connected. You would like to find ways to better manage the challenges in your life. Maybe you are someone who is:

1. Experiencing a high level of stress in your life
2. Suffering from anxiety and or depression
3. Prone to procrastinate or suffer from insomnia
4. Someone with an autoimmune disorder or someone with lots of inflammation or pain in their body
5. Simply looking to feel more at ease

This is a short list of the different ways that we can experience living with the discomfort of a dysregulated nervous system. To try and feel better, maybe you have tried things like meditation, yoga, tai chi, breathing techniques, massage therapy, acupuncture, etc. to help with these challenges; to help you grow beyond the patterns and behaviors that, for reasons that seem incomprehensible, you seem to repeat over and over again. The number of things we can try is really endless, and with all of the information available out there, it can be a real challenge to determine which techniques may be best for you. I experienced this personally, and all of my clients that I work with were experiencing the same challenge.

What I found over time is that the central nervous system is the key to effectively working on these issues and understanding why these different exercises and therapies help. By directly working with my nervous system in intentional ways, I was able to find short-term relief that eventually led to long-term success on the issues I was personally working on. In the following chapters, I will explain my approach and a number of simple exercises you can do to work with your vagus nerve to help regulate your nervous system.

The nervous system is an incredibly complex system made up of subsystems that are working to keep you alive. In order to fully understand the nervous system, you would need to invest a lot of time and effort, and in my opinion, for the majority of people, it just isn't worth it. However, when we want to achieve a specific goal, it helps to understand the subject and what we can do to achieve that specific goal. Perhaps more importantly, to understand the "why", or the mechanisms behind the activity.

What I mean by that is that if we can have a basic understanding of how our nervous system, and specifically the vagus nerve, works, we will increase our chances of success. If we understand why we are doing what we are doing and what effect this is having on our body, we can be more connected and strategic with our work. This is the goal of this book. To arm you with knowledge and exercises so you can build a plan / goal and start working towards it.

When I first realized that I had more anxiety than I was aware of, or perhaps willing to admit to myself, I started to look for ways to help myself. I found the typical things like breathing, yoga, tai chi, essential oils, etc. When I first started to use the techniques, I noticed an improvement in my anxiety and stress.

My thinking was that if I applied these techniques, I wouldn't experience anxiety anymore, and that stress would simply melt away. It is true that in the short term, I experienced less stress and anxiety. Some situations I was able to move through more gracefully than others, and some not so gracefully. However, the change was slow and felt inconsistent, so I became inconsistent with my practice and eventually stopped trying. I thought my practice would get rid of these uncomfortable feelings, but I was still experiencing higher levels of stress and anxiety than I wanted to.

I found myself repeating patterns and behaviors that were either creating the issues behind the stress and / or making the issues feel worse because of my reactions to them. To be honest, I threw in the towel more than once.

At this point in time, I started to study and learn about the nervous system and how it works. Part of this was out of necessity, as my health was starting to suffer from the stress. The other part of it was that, as I looked around, almost everyone was having a similar experience to me.

I wanted to understand "why" these exercises work. What is actually happening in my body to create the sensation of stress, anxiety, etc.? And perhaps more importantly, how can I effectively work with the nervous system to produce the outcomes I am looking for? What I have learned has been a revelation for me and has been the basis of my personal and professional work ever since.

Whenever I had success in the past working with my body, it was always built on an understanding of how the body works. When I was younger, like most boys, I wanted to be stronger and have bigger muscles. I got my first weights for training at 12 years old. I used them on and off for years, but really had no idea what I was doing.

As you can imagine, the results I achieved were less than I was hoping for. When I was about 18 years old, I started to work out more seriously and started talking to the older guys in the gym. They started to explain to me different techniques and programs that you can do to build strength and size. Things like how many repetitions to do, how much weight to use, speed of movement, which exercises are best, etc.

The interesting thing is that although there were a lot of similarities between the techniques, some were completely different and seemed to produce great results. So now I had a basic roadmap but still no understanding of why these techniques produced results.

When I really had success was when I started researching the science behind becoming strong and building muscle. I found a wealth of information that was backed by scientific studies and clearly explained the "why" behind the programs. Understanding the "why" behind the programs allowed me to be more engaged and strategic with what techniques I would use at what times. It also introduced me to the idea that nutrition was essential to having success with these programs.

At the time, I was in university, and my diet was that of a typical university student. This is not the best diet for building a healthy body and mind. However, armed with this new information, I approached my fitness program with a clear goal and a clear understanding of how the effort I was going to put in would yield the results I was looking for. As I was starting to see better results, it also helped provide me with the motivation to continue with my program.

This is what I hope to do for you with this book. I am going to give you a simplified explanation of how the nervous system works and follow that up with practical science-based methodologies to work with it.

When you finish the book, I want you to have a basic understanding of

1. What is the nervous system, and how does it work?
2. The important role the vagus nerve plays in its regulation
3. How important the nervous system is to how we perceive and interact with our world
4. How the nervous system is programmed to react in specific, predictable ways
5. How can we reprogram our nervous system to react in new ways?
6. The exercises and techniques that will allow you to work with your nervous system to achieve the results that you want

Once you have this basic understanding, you will be well-armed to start the journey of working with your nervous system. Please be patient with yourself. It takes time to learn how to work with your nervous system, and it will take some time for the changes to become lasting. I hope this book will inspire you to begin your journey!

Included with this book are videos for the exercises in Chapter 6. I have included the videos to help you learn and implement the exercises as correctly as possible. You can find the QR code to access the videos at the end of the book.

Good Luck!

Chapter 2
What is the Nervous System?

Your work with me is going to be centered on your body and your nervous system because part of the reason why we continue to act in certain ways even when we know better is because how we FEEL about things has a huge influence on our behaviors. Our feelings are in our bodies, so we need to get to know our bodies and our reactions so we can begin to work with them more consciously.

So what do I mean when I say we need to get to know our bodies and how we feel? When I say feeling, I mean being present with what is happening inside your body. This can be things like your breath, your heart rate, feelings of tension, or maybe even what is happening in your organs. Maybe you feel butterflies in your stomach or a feeling of hunger.

We also want to become more aware of the subtle sensations in your body; perhaps some parts get cold while others are warmer; maybe you have tingling in places; maybe you feel sad or angry.

And getting to know the body is a process.

At the moment, we have a certain capacity to connect with and feel what is going on in the body. We call this your neuromuscular connection, and depending on how developed it is, you will have more or less capacity to feel and control your body. We need to practice observing and moving the body consciously to develop and refine this connection. And over time, we will build a stronger connection between our brain and our body, and in doing so, we will have a better awareness of our body and what is happening inside.

It will also allow us to have greater control over the body. For example, some of the exercises I am going to teach you will feel challenging at first. Maybe you will not be able to do them exactly as I am asking you. Over time, as you build this connection, you will get better at the movements, and you will have a better ability to move and use your body how you would like to.

The more I learned and worked with the nervous system, the more I realized just how amazing of a system it is. I started to learn that the reactions that I was trying to avoid were natural and normal for MY nervous system. Although I wanted them to be different, they were the reactions that were appropriate for my nervous system and the situations I found myself in.

I learned how to observe and feel my reactions and how to interpret them in a healthy way. For example, in the past, when I was anxious, I simply wanted it to go away. I would get stuck in patterns of thinking and I didn't know how to get out of them.

I would have feelings of guilt and shame because I thought that I had evolved past the anxious feelings and believed that I should be able to do better. And this combination of getting stuck in a pattern and then feeling guilty about it somehow seemed to make it all worse. I didn't understand how the feelings actually seemed to be getting more intense, even though I was working with various techniques to help lower my anxiety. The feelings would get more intense, the thoughts would continue, and I would repeat the patterns over and over again. I needed to find a way to break this pattern!

With a little more knowledge and experience, I started to accept that my reactions were normal for me. I want you to remember this point for later: how important it is to accept our initial reactions to the world around us. Once I started to feel acceptance for my reactions, I started to make real progress with my nervous system.

The shame and guilt lessened dramatically, and I started to really understand that my nervous system was doing exactly what it was programmed to do. I also learned that to experience long-lasting change, I had to learn how to reprogram it.

One of the things that shocked me was when I learned that 90–95 percent of your brain activity is unconscious. When I say activity, I mean your habits and patterns, automatic body functions, emotions, beliefs and values, biases, and long-term memory. The reactions I was fighting against were happening as part of a program that was hidden from me. Also, as the initial reactions of my nervous system were happening as part of my unconscious programming, I couldn't control them.

This was liberating for me as I realized two things:

1. There was nothing inherently wrong with me. I simply had a nervous system that was programmed throughout my life to react in specific ways. For me, that meant a nervous system that became anxious quite easily.
2. I realized that if I wanted to live a life with more ease, I had to find a strategy to change the programming.

It's not necessary to memorize the technical terms for the central nervous system. I am including a slightly technical description of the nervous system for those of you who want to really understand the system and perhaps use this as a basis to investigate and explore further!

The nervous system of the human body is a complex network of cells and tissues that work together to control and coordinate many of the body's functions. It's similar to a massive communication network within your body, with the brain serving as the primary control center.

The nervous system is made up of two main parts: the central nervous system (CNS) and the peripheral nervous system (PNS). Each of these parts is made up of smaller subsystems. The CNS consists of the brain and spinal cord, whereas the PNS consists of all the nerves outside of the spinal column that connect the CNS to the rest of the body.

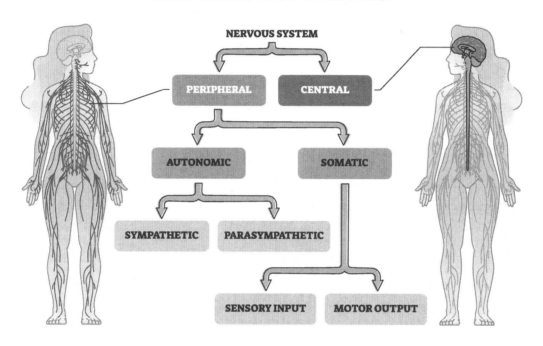

The CNS is in charge of getting information from the body's senses, such as touch, smell, sight, taste, and hearing, and figuring out what it means. It then uses this information to control the body's responses to different stimuli. For example, if you touch something that is too hot, the nerves in your hand send a signal to the spinal cord, which then relays the message to the brain. The brain processes the information and sends a signal back down to the muscles in your hand, telling them to move your hand away. All of this happens very quickly, without you even having to consciously think about it.

The brain is the center of the central nervous system and is in charge of everything, from your thoughts and emotions to your movements and bodily functions. It is an impressive organ with billions of neurons (nerve cells) that send electrical and chemical signals all over the body.

The spinal cord functions as a large "relay station," connecting the brain to the rest of the body. It's a long, thin bundle of nerves that runs down the center of the spine from the brain to your coccyx. The spinal cord is in charge of sending and receiving signals to and from the brain via bundles of nerves known as tracts.

The PNS functions as the body's communication link between the CNS and the rest of the body. It includes all of the nerves that connect your brain and spinal cord to all of the body's parts (muscles, organs, etc.). The PNS is made up of two parts: the somatic nervous system and the autonomic nervous system. This is where we will find the vagus nerve.

The somatic nervous system regulates voluntary movements and sensations like walking, talking, and feeling pressure, temperature, and pain. This system is in charge of sending information from the body's sensory receptors to the CNS and sending commands from the CNS to the skeletal muscles. Think about wanting to pick something up. Your brain registers the desire to move the muscle and sends a signal to the muscle to move. As you move your hand to pick up the object, there is sensory information flowing from the hand to the body and instructions flowing from the brain to the hand so you can successfully pick up the object.

We also have what is called the autonomic nervous system (ANS), which is part of the PNS and regulates involuntary functions such as heart rate, breathing, digestion, pupil dilation, etc. It's in charge of things you don't have to think about, like when your heart rate increases when you're scared or when you start sweating when you're nervous.

Our main focus in this book is going to be on two subcategories of the ANS called the Sympathetic and Parasympathetic nervous systems. You may have heard them referred to as "Fight or Flight" or "Rest and Digest" respectively.

This book is going to be focused on intentionally affecting these 2 aspects of the nervous system to increase or decrease the levels of excitement (fight or flight / sympathetic nervous system) and relaxation (rest and digest / parasympathetic nervous system). In essence, the sympathetic nervous system prepares the body for "fight or flight" responses by increasing heart rate and blood pressure, dilation of the pupils, and mobilization of energy reserves. It is activated in response to stress, danger, or other stimuli that necessitate an immediate response.

The parasympathetic nervous system helps the body "rest and digest" by slowing down the heart rate and breathing, making the pupils smaller, and helping digestion and getting rid of waste. It is triggered during periods of relaxation, positive social connections, rest, and digestion. The vagus nerve is part of the parasympathetic nervous system, and when it detects the right circumstances in the body and environment, it signals the parasympathetic nervous system to do its work. The result for us is a more relaxed nervous system and a feeling of being more at ease.

The parasympathetic system is where we are going to do our work! In the following chapters, we are going to dive deeper into these two systems in the ANS, and I will explain more what I mean when I say that our nervous system is programmed to react in the way it does. We will look at how it was programmed and, more importantly, how we reprogram it!

Chapter 3
What is the Vagus nerve?

Iremember a few years ago when I started to see the Vagus nerve start to pop up on my social media feeds. I saw things like "Hack your Vagus nerve and get rid of anxiety", "Reset your nervous system in 5 minutes with this simple vagus nerve exercise" and "Stimulate your vagus nerve to rid yourself of anxiety".

Obviously, it piqued my interest, and I started to investigate. What I found as I researched was that the vagus nerve is critical for our overall sense of health and well-being and our nervous system's ability to move from excited states to more relaxed states. The more I understood how the vagus nerve worked, the better I could determine if these exercises were actually going to have an impact on my vagus nerve and my overall wellbeing. I have to admit, most of these claims were greatly exaggerated, but many of the exercises did have an impact on my nervous system and, in turn, my vagus nerve!

Let's get into what the vagus nerve is and what it does so you can start working with it!

The vagus nerve is the longest nerve in the body and is actually a pair of nerves that run from the base of your brain all the way down to your abdomen. The word "Vagus", is a Latin word that means wanderer. Which is appropriate because the vagus nerve travels and makes connections

throughout the torso of the body.

As you can see from the image, the vagus nerve connects many different areas of the body to the brain.

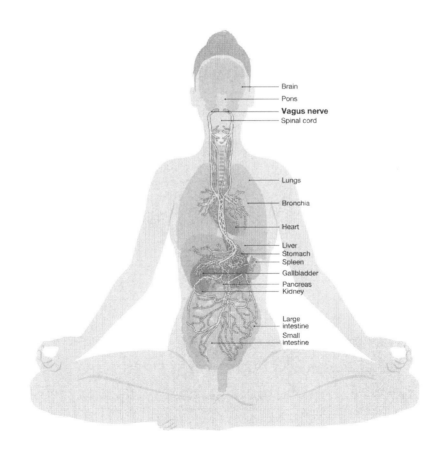

The nerve starts at the base of the brain and begins its travel down through the neck and throughout the torso, connecting with all the vital organs and various other parts of the body. It is essentially a two-way communication pathway between the brain and the different parts of the body. It allows for the regulation and coordination of many different physiological processes to maintain homeostasis and to respond to changes in our internal and external environment.

The vagus nerve is one of the pathways that allows the body to provide information to the brain about what is happening in the body (afferent pathway) and then allows the brain to send back instructions to the body (efferent pathway). For example, the vagus nerve is connected to the heart. It is monitoring the number of beats per minute, pressure in the heart, and blood pressure.

As the heart speeds up, the vagus nerve notices this and starts to stimulate the sympathetic nervous system (fight or flight) and mobilize the body's energy resources so you can deal with the challenge in front of you. This is actually exactly what you want when you are exercising or in an actual life-or-death experience. The vagus nerve will detect this and start a cascade of reactions in the body to help you survive the current moment.

Then, after the event, as the heart starts to slow down, the vagus nerve notices this and stimulates the parasympathetic nervous system (rest and digest) and starts to move the body back to a feeling of being more at ease. Now I have simplified this quite a bit, but at this stage, this is enough to know that it is the current state of the organs and the rest of the body that stimulate the vagus nerve.

These states are connected to the feelings of safety, ease, joy, stress, anxiety, fear, etc. And as we create these conditions in the body, the vagus nerve will detect them and send signals to all of the parts of the body to create the proper response. So our focus when working with the vagus nerve is to create the conditions in the nervous system as a whole, for example a slower heart rate, to allow the vagus nerve to work and move us towards states of more ease.

In addition to its involvement in the relaxation response of the body, some of the other bodily functions that the vagus nerve is involved in are:

1. Heart rate: By reducing the rate at which the heart beats, the vagus nerve aids in controlling heart rate.
2. Breathing: The vagus nerve helps to control breathing by co-ordinating the muscles that help you breathe in and out.
3. Digestion: The vagus nerve stimulates the production of digestive enzymes, boosts blood supply to the digestive organs, and regulates the passage of food through the digestive tract, all of which are important functions of the digestive system.
4. Immune system: The vagus nerve helps keep the immune system in check by limiting the release of cytokines that cause inflammation.
5. Mood: The vagus nerve controls emotions and mood and is important in helping with depression and anxiety.

6. Pain: The vagus nerve may play a role in the body's natural pain-relieving systems and can help modify pain signals.

7. Sleep: Problems sleeping may be caused by problems with the vagus nerve. This is because the vagus nerve may be involved in controlling the sleep-wake cycle.

As I mentioned earlier, we have to place working with the vagus nerve in a larger context, as there are a number of reasons why our vagus nerve is not able to regulate our nervous system back to a balanced state. We may be doing a number of things right but still not getting the results we want.

Here are some of the common things that can affect the health and function of the vagus nerve. Some of them I address in this book, but I wanted to give you a more complete list as you may want to investigate some of the other areas if they apply to you.

1. Chronic Stress: Stress that lasts for a long time can keep the sympathetic nervous system active, which can reduce the activity of the vagus nerve and make it less able to control how the body works.

2. Poor Sleep: Insomnia and sleep apnea can mess up the body's natural circadian cycle and lead to problems with the autonomic nervous system, including problems with the vagus nerve.

3. Sedentary Lifestyle: If you don't move around much, your heart may not work as well, which can hurt the vagus nerve by cutting off blood flow and oxygen to nerve cells.

4. Poor gut health: The vagus nerve and the gut are linked, and conditions like irritable bowel syndrome (IBS), chronic inflammation, or abnormalities in the gut microbiota can effect the activity of the vagus nerve.

5. Some medication: Medications that can interfere with the vagus nerve's ability to control body activities include antipsychotics, blood pressure medicines, and antidepressants.

As you can see, the vagus nerve plays a very important role in our mental and physical health. As you learn how to engage and work with your vagus nerve, you will discover that you can have a much greater influence on your nervous system than you may have thought possible.

Chapter 4
Neuroplasticity: How We Change Our Nervous System

*"Do the best you can until you know better.
Then when you know better, do better."*

MAYA ANGELOU

Neuroplasticity is a term that simply means that the nervous system (remember, the brain is included in the nervous system) is capable of changing. In truth, it is constantly changing as we have experiences in our lives. When we have new experiences, our nervous system changes to capture the new experience and subtly changes our program.

Our challenge is that our nervous system is programmed and has a set of patterns that we unconsciously repeat. This means that the majority of our experiences will be the same as past experiences, so although our nervous system is capable of changing throughout our lives, we reinforce our programming by repeating these patterns.

If you have been observing your thoughts and patterns over time, you will have seen certain patterns of thinking. Just like we have conditioned patterns in our minds, we also have conditioned patterns in our bodies. We are conditioned to feel certain ways in certain situations, and these feelings usually lead us to think the same way and, in turn, make the same decisions.

As you gain more experience with the exercises in the book, you are going to shine a spotlight on these patterns and learn how to recondition our nervous systems and bodies so we can start to change these programs. You are going to build new programs that will allow you to live with more ease.

I think it's helpful to understand what we mean by conditioning or programming. I remember when I first started to study the brain and nervous system, I was shocked to learn that the majority of our programming happens before we are 8 years old and that 90–95 percent of the activity in our minds is below the level of our consciousness. I want you to think about that for a moment.

On average, we have about 60,000 thoughts a day, and 90–95 percent are the same as yesterday. This means that the majority of our reactions, thoughts, patterns, habits, and behaviors are happening automatically. The challenge is that we can't see our subconscious thoughts in real time. But with practice, we will begin to feel the reactions in our bodies in real time. This is why the body is so important in our process of getting to know ourselves.

The body has also been conditioned to react to our subconscious mind. The typical flow of energy in the nervous system is that our senses are monitoring our internal and external environments and informing our nervous system what is happening. After our subconscious mind has gathered the information about what is happening in and around us, the information flows to a part of our brain that is responsible for creating how we feel in our body.

This area of the brain works with the vagus nerve to create a feeling in the body. Remember that this feeling is highly influential in how we will eventually act, so we need to have clarity on how we feel!

Our first conscious experience of our subconscious programming is actually a feeling in the body. We then typically try to make sense of that feeling with our conscious mind by creating a story that allows us to logically make sense of our world. That story is going to be flavored by how we feel. What do I mean by flavoring? Our nervous system will always be biased toward information that matches the state we are in. So when we are in a negative state, we will focus on and experience things in a more negative light. The good news is that this holds true for positive states as well.

So what does this really mean for us? If our minds and bodies have been conditioned to behave in predictable patterns that we repeat over and over again, How do we break or change the programming?

The programming, or conditioning, that we have is physically built into us. The structure in our brain, the tone in our nervous system, the chemical balance in our body, our postures, etc. are all part of our conditioning. So in order to change our conditioning, we need to physically change our brain, our nervous system, and how it responds to the world.

The great news is that our bodies and our nervous system are adaptable. That means that just like your muscles, we can exercise our nervous system to change it! How do we do this? Through new and meaningful experiences. The typical unconscious process is as follows: I want to point out that the following process can also start with a thought, but as we are working with the body here, let's start with a feeling. It essentially is like this; you have an experience and you feel a certain way about it.

Depending on how we feel, our bias in the nervous system will lead us to interpret and think about the event in a way that is in alignment with that feeling. You will then need to make a decision, which in turn leads you to take an action that will result in you having an experience.

Remember that it is the experiences in our lives that change our nervous systems and bodies. So if we are in this process unconsciously, we typically feel the same way most of the time. What I mean is that we have patterns of how we feel, so we have the same types of thoughts, which lead to the same actions, which lead to the same experiences, which lead to strengthening our existing patterns. And remember that 90–95 percent of this process is happening unconsciously, so we need to change the system so that our natural responses are in alignment with how we want to live.

I say naturally because, at first, these changes we start to make will not feel natural. In fact, they will probably feel pretty uncomfortable. One of the main purposes of our nervous system is to keep us alive. Our nervous system and mind have a survival strategy that has kept you alive so far, so there will be resistance to stepping outside of that strategy.

This means that until we have reprogrammed our nervous system to one that we are happy with, we have to be consciously involved and really aware of ourselves. Aware of how we are feeling, thinking, and acting. In essence, getting to know our unconscious patterns.

With this awareness, we will make new choices that will lead to new experiences that will, over time, change our nervous system. Once it has been changed, we will have a new natural reaction within our nervous system.

Chapter 5
Polyvagal Theory

I wanted to put PolyVagal Theory in this book because it has helped me and my clients in so many ways. Polyvagal Theory describes how our nervous system influences our emotions and behavior. Dr. Stephen Porges first presented the theory in 1994, and it has since undergone several revisions and refinements.

Polyvagal Theory can be traced back to Dr. Porges's earlier research on how the ANS controls social behavior. Porges studied how animals' bodies react to stress in the 1970s. He found that the ANS is a key factor in deciding whether an animal will fight, run away, or freeze when it thinks it is in danger.

Earlier in the book, we spoke about the two systems we are going to be working with in our exercises. Polyvagal theory was eye-opening for me as it introduced me to a third aspect of our nervous system that we can use to regulate it. According to Polyvagal Theory, our nervous system is divided into three parts that work together to help us respond to various situations.

The first part is known as the "sympathetic" or "fight-or-flight" response, and it allows us to react quickly to danger. It causes our hearts to race and prepares us to either fight or flee the danger.

The second part is known as the "parasympathetic" or "rest and digest" response, and it assists us in relaxing and recovering after the danger has passed. It lowers our heart rate and makes us feel more relaxed.

The third component is known as the "social engagement system." This section teaches us how to interact with others in a safe and effective manner. It facilitates communication and the formation of social bonds.

These three parts of our nervous system interact in a specific order, according to Polyvagal Theory. First, we respond to danger by engaging in "fight or flight." If the threat has passed, we switch to the "rest and digest" response to unwind. Finally, if we feel safe and calm, we engage in "social engagement" with others.

Polyvagal Theory is important because it explains how our bodies and emotions are linked. It also explains how trauma and stress can affect our nervous system and ability to connect with others. Understanding how our nervous system works allows us to better manage our emotions and respond to situations.

In the past few years, Polyvagal Theory has continued to grow as researchers have looked into new parts of the autonomic nervous system (ANS) and how they relate to social interaction and controlling emotions. It is one of the best-known and most important theories in the field of psychophysiology right now. Deb Dana is one of the leading experts in this field, and her book "PolyVagal Theory in Therapy" helps us understand how we can use this scientific theory to examine and understand our patterns.

The exercises in this book are designed to teach you how to regulate a dysregulated nervous system once it has been triggered. But wouldn't it be even better if you could identify and remove some of the triggers before they affected you? This is why I am including the polyvagal theory for you. It isn't an exercise in the typical sense. But it will help you identify the events and patterns in your life that are affecting your nervous system in negative and positive ways. Once you have identified them, you can work to address the things that are impacting your nervous system in a negative way and focus more of your time and effort on the things that are affecting your nervous system in a positive way.

Polyvagal Theory is made up of three principles that are important to understand.

1. Hierarchy or Polyvagal Ladder
2. Neuroception
3. Co-Regulation

The first principle says that energy moves in predictable ways that depend on how safe we feel or how dangerous we think something is. Deb Dana has called this movement of energy the Poly-Vagal Ladder.

At the top of the ladder, we have what we call the social engagement system. This system is active when all is well in our lives, we are feeling safe, and we have deep and meaningful connections with the people in our lives. Essentially, things are going well.

This state is called "Safe and Social". Now, when something goes "wrong", we would say we move down the ladder to a fight or flight state. And when we do this, the body starts to dump energy into the nervous system and the body in general. This makes sense because we need energy so we can attend to whatever problem or challenge is in front of us. Ideally, we use this energy, take care of the problem, and move back up the ladder.

However, if we can't fix the problem, or if the problem has been in our lives for so long that it starts to feel like we can't fix it, we move down the ladder even more into what's called shutdown, and the nervous system starts to take energy out of the system. It makes sense, right? If you can't take any meaningful action to fix the issue, why waste energy? The body starts to conserve energy so that when the threat is gone, or at least manageable, you will have energy to deal with it. We would then move back up to fight or flight and ideally use this energy to take care of the problem, then move back to safe and social.

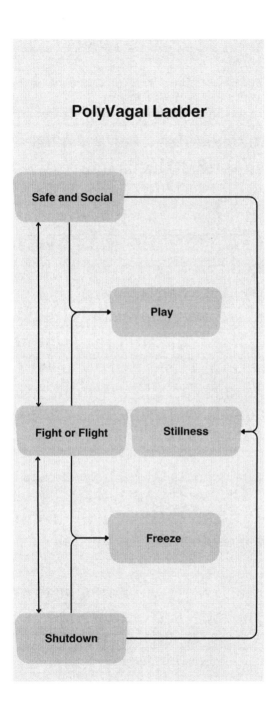

I want to make a very important point here. We are not trying to train our nervous systems to be nonreactive. This movement of energy up and down the ladder is an amazing process that helps to keep us alive.

We don't want to avoid reactions in our system! If there is danger, we want our body to recognize it so we can have the energy to deal with it. It's not a bad thing to feel a bit of pressure when you have a project due, for example. This energy helps us complete things, and we don't want to numb ourselves to these feelings. In fact, it is just the opposite. We want to get curious about them and get to know them really well.

I introduced you to the three main states that help us understand the movement of energy. We actually have three more states that we can find ourselves in. Don't worry; as you start to pay attention to your patterns and view them through the lens of Polyvagal Theory, these states will start to become very clear and familiar to you.

That makes a total of six states we are going to learn. Let's go over the three main states, and then we will dive into the three other states. Let's start with the three main ones.

At the top of the ladder, we have the social engagement system. It can also be called the safe and social state. This system is active when we feel safe and secure in our lives. If you look at the picture in Chapter 3, the portion of the nerve that is between the heart and the head will be active when we are in this state. When this portion of the nerve is active and functioning well, we will move into a socially engaged state, and our focus will shift to relationships and connection.

So how else can we know if we are in this state? Well, when we are in this state, our heart beats at a normal pace, our breathing is full, we are able to tune into conversations with friends and block out distracting noises, and the structure of our ears actually changes so we can better focus on individual voices and block out background noises.

Essentially, we have the desire and urge to connect to the world. We will also find that in our lives it will be easier to be organized, we will follow through with plans we make, we will take care of ourselves, and we will make time to play. We enjoy being with others, we feel productive, and we have a good balance in our lives. We will have better digestion, a healthier immune system, sleep better, and generally just feel better! When this part of the nerve is activated, we will naturally feel this way.

When we start to experience challenges in our lives, the nervous system will mobilize energy, activate the nervous system, and move us down the ladder to the fight or flight state. Typically, if the danger is not too great, the system releases a little energy, and we will choose flight. If the danger is greater, we will mobilize more energy in order to fight.

We have to remember that the main purpose of this system is to keep us alive. So, we want a system that will mobilize energy when necessary. The challenges that we want to work on are when we mobilize energy when there isn't actually a threat, when we mobilize too much energy for the challenge in front of us, or if we become "stuck" in a chronic state of activation.

So how do we know we are in the fight or flight state? We start to feel uneasy; we may call this an anxious feeling, and feelings of anger are common in this state. The world around us feels chaotic and dangerous—maybe a little bit too much.

There are actual physical changes that take place in our body when we are in fight or flight. Our vision changes, so it is actually more difficult to see the emotional states in others faces. We will see normal facial expressions as possible cues of danger, and your body is going to react. It also restricts blood flow to the brain and makes critical thinking and remembering things more difficult.

We will have challenges in our relationships as we approach situations not looking for a solution that benefits both parties, but rather looking for conflict and definitely looking to win. Our sense of the world starts to narrow; we feel separated from others, and we become more focused on ourselves and how to survive. Social harmony and harmony in our relationships are not at the top of our priorities.

These states work well in certain situations, but we are meant to be in them for short periods of time. When our body's fight-or-flight system is active, our body prioritizes survival over health. For short periods of time, this is not a problem, but if we are in these states too often or stay in them too long, our health will start to suffer.

Some of the health issues that come from being in fight or flight mode for too long include heart disease, weight gain, headaches, and chronic neck, shoulder, and back tension. It is more difficult for us to sleep deeply so that we can feel rested in the morning, and over time our immune system starts to function at a reduced capacity.

You can see this vicious circle in modern society. People get stuck in fight or flight and can't slow down to start taking care of themselves. These are the people you know who literally can't sit still for moments. They have to be moving, or watching TV, or on their phones, or really doing anything at all, so they don't have to slow down and feel this energy running through them.

The bottom rung on the ladder is called the shutdown state, and we enter this state when we feel trapped. The immediate danger is too much for our systems to handle, or the danger we have in our lives has persisted for so long that we don't see a way out. When we find ourselves in an environment like this, our nervous system will want to conserve energy and start to take energy away from us.

When we are in this state, we feel hopeless, alone with despair, abandoned. We are going to be tired, and it will be difficult to think or act, and we are going to feel alone and lost. We will have brain fog and memory problems, and a typical strategy for someone in shutdown is to isolate themselves because they have no energy to do anything.

People who are in chronic states of shutdown can start to have the following health problems: Things like chronic fatigue, fibromyalgia, stomach problems, low blood pressure, type 2 diabetes, and weight gain. When we are removing energy from the system, we call this immobilization, and a typical example of this would be burnout.

In our society today, we place a high value on people who work hard. People who worked crazy hours were frequently the heroes in my corporate days. They never stopped! They would take on project after project and do as much as they could to get ahead. And even those who weren't trying to work that hard and get to the top were typically being driven by their bosses to deliver. The environment felt a lot more like one of competition than cooperation.

This type of environment continuously activates the fight-or-flight system. Remember that our systems are built to adapt to stresses for short periods of time. We will create energy to deal with problems, and then ideally we will move back to a safe and social state. But in corporate culture, the environment is typically not one that feels safe and social. So our workplace becomes one of our main stressors, and if we stay in a fight or flight state for too long or go there too often, our bodies will start to go into shutdown.

Shutdown can start by simply feeling that you are tired all the time. Your body has been trying to support you, but it is starting to tell you it is reaching its limits. It is trying to ask you to rest, and if you don't listen, it may force you to rest. If you continue to ignore the body's warnings, you may go into full shutdown and go into "burnout".

This is so damaging to the body that, on average, it takes about

8–12 months of rest to repair your nervous system enough so you start to feel normal again. To get back to an optimal state, this often takes years, so we need to listen to our bodies!

These are the three main states in PolyVagal theory, and there are also three "mixed" states, for a total of six states. The first three states are a good place to start to understand the movement of energy through your nervous system as you live your life. As you get more familiar with these main states, you should start to explore the three mixed states more as well.

The first mixed state is called Play. This state happens when we have the social engagement system active (brain-heart connection) and the fight-or-flight system activated. In other words, we feel the urge or necessity to do something, so we create energy, but the environment is safe, so you enter the state of play.

Sports are a great example of this. We are competing, but there are a set of rules that everyone is following, and this provides a safe container for us to play in. As long as the heart-brain part of the vagus nerve is activated, the activity will have a safe and fun feeling. If during the activity we perceive a cue of danger—maybe someone breaks one of the rules—we will lose the tone in the heart-brain part of the vagus nerve and move into the pure state of fight or flight. This is where we will probably start to see conflict between the players.

This is very common among kids playing a game. The group is playing, and there is a lot of laughing and fun. At one moment, one of the players breaks one of the rules, and suddenly the energy between the players changes. The smiling faces may disappear, and the fun competition turns into conflict.

The second mixed state is called stillness. It is a combination of safe / social, and shutdown states. So in other words, we are feeling safe, and the body starts to remove energy from the system as it is not needed at this time. We enter this state when we do things like meditate, sit and breathe, or when we are in a pleasant and safe environment and we are not really doing anything.

Think about lying on a beach, sitting in a forest, or sitting in silence with a friend. Common experiences in this state are that we are able to understand and feel the connection between people. It is easier for us to see the big picture of things. We would describe ourselves as happy, calm, and at peace, and we also have a deeper sense of gratitude.

The last state is called freeze, and although it is similar to shutdown, it is uniquely different. Freeze state occurs when we mix the states of fight or flight with shutdown. A good way to differentiate between the two is that shutdown has the feeling of going limp, whereas freeze is associated with stiffening the body. In the freeze state, we have a buildup of fight and flight energy and the urge to use that energy, but at the same time, the body is removing our energy and urging us to stay still.

Panic and phobias are two of the most common examples of this. We are highly charged with energy and feel the immediate urge to act, but we can't because our body is also removing energy at the same time. If you want to see a very clear example of shutdown, do a Google search for people passing out on rollercoasters.

You can see the fear in them, and when the fear becomes too much for their system to handle, all energy is removed from the body and they pass out. If you want to see what freeze looks like, do a search for fainting goats. When they get scared, their bodies go stiff, they can't move, and they fall down. This will give you a good sense of the difference between these two states.

The second principle in Polyvagal Theory is called neuroception. This term refers to the way our nervous system detects and responds to cues of safety or danger in our environment. This process happens automatically and outside of our conscious awareness, and it affects our emotional and physiological responses.

Healthy neuroception is when our nervous system accurately detects cues of safety or danger in our environment and responds appropriately. For example, if we are walking alone at night and hear a loud noise, our nervous system will quickly detect this as a potential danger and activate our "fight or flight" response, preparing us to either run away or defend ourselves.

We could call our neuroception unhealthy if our nervous system either overreacts or underreacts to cues of safety or danger. For example, if we have been through a traumatic event in the past, our nervous system may be overly sensitive to certain triggers that remind us of the event. This can make us feel anxious or panicked even when the situation is safe. If we've been under constant stress or haven't been cared for, our nervous system may become hypoactive. This means that it doesn't react as strongly to signs of safety or danger, making us feel numb or disconnected from our surroundings.

By understanding the different states and types of neuroception within the framework of Polyvagal Theory, you will be able to better understand how your nervous system responds to your environment and come up with ways to promote healthy neuroception and control our emotional and physical responses. As I mentioned before, it is important to learn how to regulate your nervous system into healthier states, but even better is to learn how your nervous system is reacting to the world around you and begin to live in a way that triggers your system less.

The third principle in Polyvagal Theory is called co-regulation. In our exercises, we will focus on methods to self regulate, but as you become more familiar with this theory, you will start to identify external things that help us move back up the ladder. This will be other people, places, sounds, smells, etc. that will help with co-regulation.

For me, this is the most important and powerful aspect of Porges work. We are social creatures and have an innate longing for connection with other beings. This isn›t just other humans. Animals and nature are also powerful co-regulators. Everyone who has a pet at home knows how nice it feels when you arrive at home and are greeted with love and affection. Pets are great co-regulators as we feel safe with them, so we can let our defenses down and open up fully. One of my strategies to co-regulate is to lay down on the floor and cuddle or play with my dogs when I get home. Nature is also a powerful co-regulator.

The fresh air, freedom, and beauty of nature can help bring you back to a state of social engagement very easily. Work to find what yours are and make the effort to add them to your lives!

Once you are familiar with the states and start to observe how energy moves through your system on a daily basis, you can use the following approach designed by Deb Dana to start to reprogram your nervous system.

The four steps we have to follow are:

1. Recognize the state your nervous system is in.
2. Accept the response.
3. Regulate (using the exercises in the book) or co-regulate (using external things like people, pets, and nature) into a safe and social state.
4. Re-story

#1: Recognize the state your nervous system is in.

The first step in the process is to recognize what state we are in. In order to do that, we have to become more skilled at becoming aware of our daily movements up and down the ladder. I will keep reminding you that we want our nervous system to react to our environment. We do not want to try and get rid of our reactions because they are necessary. What we want to do is work with the vagus nerve and build resilience and the ability for our body to effectively regulate itself in and out of states.

But in order to do that, we need to get to know our patterns better. Eventually, I hope you befriend your nervous system and start to feel awe and gratitude for this amazing part of your body that has helped keep you alive your entire life.

So how do we increase our awareness of our states? The first step, once you have familiarized yourself with the different states within polyvagal theory, is to start being a more conscious observer of our lives. You should start paying attention to how your body feels in certain situations.

We also need to pay attention to the types of thoughts that arise when we are in these states. It's quite normal that, as you develop your skill in observing your body, it is easier to catch your thoughts than to feel the reaction in your body. For example, you may notice that your thoughts are conflictive in nature. Maybe you are imagining an argument with someone or having a conflict with them. This is a pretty good sign that our nervous system is in a state of fight or flight.

Two useful sayings you can remember to help you with this are "Story Follows State" or "Meaning Follows Feeling". What this means is that, depending on the state of our nervous system, we will perceive what is happening through the lens of that state. If we are in a fight or flight state, the stories we create will have a foundation of danger or conflict.

Conversely, if we experience the same situation in a safe and social state our perception of the event will be different. It will be more collaborative and take the other person's needs into consideration. We are meaning-making machines, and the states of our nervous systems will determine the flavor of the stories we create. I hope this illustrates why it is important to work on increasing our awareness of our different states and the accompanying feelings and thoughts that accompany them. For me to really know who I am, I need clarity on my mental, physical, and emotional states. By intimately knowing all three, I will start to know who I really am!

You can start to build a map of your states and the things that move you up and down the ladder. For the states that we would associate as being more positive (Safe and Social, Play, Stillness), we will begin to notice and document the things that make us feel safe, happy, full of energy and life, creative, playful, curious, emotional (in a happy way), and that inspire us and provide us a sense of gratitude.

One of the best clues as to what really is important to me are the kinds of things that make you emotional in a positive way. For example, maybe when you watch videos of people accomplishing their goals, or videos of people helping other people, you get emotional or maybe even get goose bumps. Maybe it's videos of kids playing together or people being reunited after some time apart. Pay close attention to these situations because your emotional response tells you that there is something important for you to see here.

As you make your list, it is important to focus on the little things just as much as the big things. The big things are usually pretty obvious and easy to identify. However, the smaller things can also have a big influence on our lives, which is why it is important to become aware of them as well. We don't need to identify everything right away, just keep paying attention and you will continue to observe new things and gain greater clarity on things you have already found!

For the states that we consider more negative (Fight, Flight, Shutdown and Freeze) we want to start noticing the things that trigger us to move down the ladder. So how do I know I have been triggered? Well, some of the things you may notice in your body are a sense of anxiety, tightening in your neck, chest, shoulders, and back, a change in breath; you might find yourself holding your breath, a quickening of your heart rate, a sudden lack of energy, a lack of motivation, and also your thoughts will change to be more conflictive or victim-type thinking.

Your list will most likely start with the bigger things, but as you get more connected with your body, you will become more aware of the smaller triggers. Eventually you will become very attuned to your system and be able to observe, accompany, and regulate your reactions in a more conscious way!

The outcome of these lists is not to try and control everything in your life so you don't experience negative states. Rather, it is to identify the "good" and the "bad", the things that move us up the ladder and the things that move us down the ladder.

From here, you can begin to make changes in your life so that your environment starts to feel safer and there are fewer cues of danger. Maybe you notice that on the days you hit the snooze button a few times too many, you feel stressed as soon as you start your day because you are already behind schedule. Your chances of being late for work are now much higher. So, you could decide to go to bed 30 minutes earlier and not hit your snooze button. If you find that getting out of bed earlier results in you not feeling stressed out every morning, that is a relatively easy change that starts each one of your days off higher on the ladder.

Simple things like this can have a profound impact on us. So pay attention, you may have some simple things you can change that will start to have a major impact on you.

#2: Respect the survival response of your system.

If we remember how our nervous system works, it becomes clear why we must accept and surrender to our reactions. If we remember how energy moves through the nervous system according to the polyvagal ladder, it may start with everything being good, and then our nervous system perceives a cue that something is wrong.

Basically, something is happening that we are not in agreement with—so our nervous system mobilizes energy (fight or flight) so we can respond with an action to resolve the issue. This is what our system is supposed to do. But what happens when we are not in agreement with how our body is responding? For example, you just learned some unpleasant news and are experiencing anxiety.

Now you don't like the feeling of being anxious and want it to go away. Our physical response (which is the feeling of anxiety) to a potential threat has now also become a threat. The anxiety itself has become a threat because we are not accepting it, so that tells our nervous system we need to mobilize more energy to deal with this problem. As we mobilize energy, we feel the sensation more intensely and most likely will reject it more, so the body produces more energy to deal with the problem.

You can see where this is going. In the body, when we have a response to an external stimulus, the initial response lasts less than 2 minutes. The way that we prolong the feeling and intensify it is by resisting it or engaging with it by creating a story around it.

I often get asked the question "What does letting go, surrendering, and accepting really mean?". How do I practically accept, surrender to, or let go of something like anger or sadness? By understanding how energy moves through the nervous system, it is clear that letting go actually means accepting how your nervous system is reacting to whatever is happening.

We allow the feeling to exist in the body and make a more concerted effort to breathe in a way that will help regulate the nervous system. We observe the thoughts that arise, recognize that they are being influenced by the state of my body, and do our best not to engage with them. Our mind doesn't really know the difference between our imagination and our reality. So if we are triggered by something, our first experience is a feeling in the body.

Then our conscious mind creates a story that makes sense of the feeling. Sometimes this story is right, and sometimes it isn't. But that's besides the point. There is a feedback loop in the body as the body and mind work together. It looks like this: How we feel influences how we think, and how we think influences how we feel. So if I am triggered by something and this may trigger a dialogue in my head. If I don't notice, and engage with the stories that are being created, I will reinforce and potentially increase the feeling in my body, and in turn, that feeling will reinforce our story.

This will ensure I stay in this state longer than is necessary. The longer I stay in these states, the more I condition my body to want to be in and return to these states. I start to create what is, in essence, a bias or addiction toward certain states. So when we repeat and tell our stories over and over again, we relive these emotional states, recondition our bodies to them, and reinforce our thought patterns. This isn't to say we shouldn't tell stories about our lives, but we should do it in a more conscious way and perhaps begin to tell our more positive and uplifting stories more often than our stories of our challenges and problems.

This step is also very important in building a greater level of resilience in our nervous system. Our level of resiliency speaks to our ability to allow, accept, and observe reactions in our nervous system. Someone with a high level of resiliency can have a lot of energy moving through their system and still function at a high level.

On the other hand, someone who isn't very resilient will have trouble dealing with even small problems. We may also be resilient in different ways. Some of us will be great at dealing with serious situations in our lives but really struggle with the day-to-day stresses. Others can handle the day-to-day stresses but really struggle with the bigger things in life. Our map will help us learn how resilient we are and in what areas of our lives.

There is a concept in polyvagal theory called the vagal brake. It is a part of the vagus nerve that controls our heart rate, and we can think of it as something that influences how much energy moves into or out of our system. It also affects how fast and for how long this happens. When our vagal brake is functioning well, it helps us react in a way appropriate for the situation and will help us regulate ourselves into a more balanced state.

One of our exercises will work on improving the function of our vagal brake!

#3: Regulate or co-regulate into a ventral vagal state.

This may sound a little bit contradictory to rule number 2. Aren't we rejecting our response if we try to change our state? If I feel a certain way, but I want to change it, aren't I rejecting my response?

The answer is that it all has to do with how we approach our responses and the intent behind our actions. If we get curious about our responses and get good at observing them and our thoughts, we will have achieved step #1. By not engaging, we will have allowed the initial response in the body to happen freely, and as we observe and do not engage, we should start to move up the ladder a little. We will feel that the intensity of our reaction has decreased and that our nervous system is climbing the ladder. Now we have achieved step #2. At this stage, it is appropriate to work with the nervous system and accompany it as we move further up the ladder.

Think of the following example: A friend calls you and asks if he can come over to talk because he is having some sort of problem. When he arrives, he starts to explain his problem to you and becomes emotional, starting to cry. Now which approach makes more sense? Allow your friend to cry, express himself, and discharge a little of his energy before you ask if he needs any help. Or when he starts to cry, should you jump in and tell him crying isn´t the right reaction, that it's not going to help, and start to tell him how to fix his problem? Obviously, the first one.

A lot of the time, we don't even need to try to fix the problem. Simply being an observer of the energy allows it to dissipate to a level where we can start to fix the issue. The same is true with ourselves. The subtleness of it has to do with timing and intent. Come back to the example with your friend. If you simply placed your hand on his leg and looked into his eyes as he spoke, you are not trying to fix the problem. You are simply being with him and reassuring him that everything will be OK.

As we observe our reactions, we can use our breath and affirming thoughts or statements to accompany ourselves as we accept and allow our reactions to take place, and then allow our nervous system to start to regulate itself. Now, it isn't always this simple. Sometimes we will be in a situation that is quite difficult.

And a reminder that one of the most important concepts around safety is that, as humans, we have an ingrained desire for and need for connection. We need to develop deep and meaningful connections in order to feel safe in our lives. So when breathing isn't working to regulate your state, please go and connect with other human beings. It is the fastest and most effective way to co-regulate yourself back up the ladder!

And if you think about it, you have had countless experiences like this. Maybe you had a bad day and, on your way home, bumped into a good friend. You shared some smiles and laughs, and when you left that person, you probably noticed that you were happier and felt better!

#4: Re-Story

When we are in one of the lower states on the ladder, our main preoccupation is survival. When we are in survival mode, we become more self-centered, and the perception of our events will most likely be skewed. We tend to view our experiences from more of a victim standpoint, and we tend to disempower ourselves by blaming others.

This is a natural process based on our state. Remember, story follows state. If we follow the first three steps and are able to regulate or co-regulate ourselves back to a safe and social state, our perception of the event will change, and in turn, the story we create. In time, we will naturally create stories that more accurately reflect the real happenings of the event. We will be more willing to look at how our actions contributed to the event, and with this clarity, hopefully we will learn how to not repeat the pattern.

Before we finish the theory, I want to recap a few important points and give you some things to think about to keep moving forward on your journey with your body. Remember, this is just a start, and the journey with your body is for the rest of your life! Polyvagal Theory is one way in which we can help to increase our mental and physical wellness, but we have to consider other things as well.

So, a few rules to remember:

1. Awareness is the key! If we aren't aware of something, we can't change it.
2. Our nervous system is designed to keep us alive, and our responses are part of our conditioning. So the responses we have are correct for how we are currently programmed. The key to changing them is to get good at observing them and learning how to accept them.
3. We can't fake it. We need to learn to recognize and accept our responses. Our bodies will not believe our minds.
4. Connection is key! Learning how to regulate our nervous system is very important and helps us to build resiliency, but to reach the top rung of the ladder, we need to have deep and meaningful connections with others and with life.
5. It's a journey...work hard and be patient. We need to give our nervous systems and bodies time to adapt to the new person we are trying to be. In the meantime, while our body is in our old reality and our conscious mind is trying to build our new

reality, we will need to work hard to consciously direct our actions and decisions. If you feel this approach is not giving you fast enough results, stick with it. If you want to, you can start to investigate how things like diet, exercise, posture, sleep quality, and hydration can affect the performance of your nervous system and vagus nerve. What most people experience as they start this process is that it is not a linear path from where you are to where you want to be. You will have successes and setbacks. You will handle some situations with ease and other situations may affect you a great deal. Remember, that this is a process and that it takes time to reshape your nervous system! So when you feel like you have had a setback, remember that by sticking to your exercises, over time you will have success. Keep your focus on the process and over time you will get the results you want.

6. Be gentle on yourself. You are doing your best!

Chapter 6
Exercises

Disclaimer: Before beginning any new exercise program, it is important to consult with your healthcare provider, especially if you have any underlying health conditions or injuries. The information in this book is provided solely for educational purposes and is not intended to be medical advice. Before beginning any new exercise program or making any changes to your current exercise routine, always consult with your healthcare provider. If you experience any pain, discomfort, or other symptoms while practicing these exercises, you should immediately stop and seek medical attention.

I have included a basic description for all of the exercises, but I would recommend you view the videos to ensure you are doing them as correctly as possible. The videos can be found by scanning the QR code at the end of the book. Good Luck!

Sleep

I know sleeping isn't really an exercise, but I wanted to include it as sleep is one of the fundamental things we have to get better at if we want to have success working with our nervous system and feeling more at ease. You have all experienced what it is like when you are not sleeping well. You feel groggy, and it is difficult to focus and be motivated to take on life. We are also often more grumpy or reactive to the world around us. Conversely, when you get a great sleep, you are often in a much better mood, better able to focus and achieve things during your waking hours, and things that typically may stress you out will have less impact on you.

This is because sleep is essential for maintaining a healthy nervous system. When we sleep, our brain has a chance to rest, repair, and recharge, allowing us to function optimally during the day. Sleep is especially important for regulating stress and our emotional reactions to stress.

While we sleep, our brains process and store memories and feelings. This helps us make sense of our lives and deal with stress. This process is critical for preventing stress buildup, which can lead to chronic stress and other health issues.

Sleep is also important because it helps control the autonomic nervous system. This system controls many of the body's automatic functions, like breathing, digestion, and heart rate. When we sleep, our bodies relax, which turns on the parasympathetic part of the nervous system. This aids in the reduction of stress hormones such as cortisol and adrenaline while also promoting a sense of calm.

Inadequate or poor quality sleep, on the other hand, can be harmful to the nervous system. Chronic sleep deprivation has been linked to a variety of health issues, including depression, anxiety, and cognitive impairment. Inadequate sleep can also cause autonomic nervous system dysregulation, which can lead to increased stress and decreased resilience to stress.

If you find that when you get up in the morning, you don't feel rested, then I would suggest you start with the following suggestions to help you sleep better. Many of us can lay down at night, fall asleep, and stay asleep for 8 hours and still wake up feeling tired and groggy. Just because you have slept all night does not mean you are getting the benefits of a deep and restful sleep.

To start working towards having a better night's sleep, please try incorporating some or all of these things into your daily routine.

1. Timing: We have a rhythm in our body called the circadian rhythm. This is essentially a clock in our brain that determines when we want to be sleepy and when we want to be awake. This clock starts in the morning with a release of cortisol, and about 12 to 14 hours later, your body will release melatonin, and you will start to feel sleepy. The timing of these two different states is determined by light, specifically sunlight. When you wake up in the morning and expose yourself to light, the clock starts. What happens is that the body releases cortisol, and this is what makes you feel more alert and awake. The

quality of the light (sunlight) has a dramatic effect on whether that surge of energy is enough to properly set your circadian rhythm. Artificial light will produce a smaller release, so you will start to feel sleepier earlier in the day, and your circadian rhythm will be affected. You may have heard of cortisol as the stress hormone. Although this is true, this release of cortisol in the morning is part of a healthy and well-functioning nervous system. What this means for you is that as soon as possible after waking up, get to a window or, even better, get outside for 5 minutes and allow sunlight to enter your eyes. With consistency, this will help you strengthen your circadian rhythm so your body can keep you awake and alert all day and allow you to get a deep night's sleep.

2. Relaxation: The connection between our wakeful and sleeping hours is very important. When my life is more stressful, I find that although I sleep all night, I don't wake up as well rested. That is because the hormones and neurotransmitters that are in my body when I am stressed don't allow me to enter as deeply into a restful state. I have given you a number of exercises to help you balance your nervous system, and please choose one of them to practice before bed. My personal choice is the physiological sigh. And sometimes I will combine this with music I like.

3. Light: Even small amounts of light in your bedroom can affect your quality of sleep because light is a powerful cue that influences our sleep-wake cycle. As I said, light makes our bodies make the hormone cortisol, which wakes us up, and stops our brains from making the hormone melatonin, which makes us sleepy. So, even small amounts of light in your bedroom can stop your body from making its own melatonin, which makes

it hard to fall asleep and stay asleep all night. So if it is possible, make your bedroom as dark as possible and avoid exposing yourself to light during the night. Consider using a sleeping mask if it is not possible to make your bedroom very dark.

4. Food: When you go to sleep, your body wants to rest and repair itself. To do this, it needs to use the resources available to complete the work. However, if your body is trying to digest a stomach full of food, energy that could be used to repair your body will be used on digestion. Also, as your body is actively digesting your food, it will not be able to enter as deep a state of rest. So it is best to avoid eating within 2-3 hours of going to bed.

5. Caffeine: As we all know, caffeine is an amazing stimulant that helps us stay alert and awake. What you may not know is that caffeine has a half-life of approximately 6 hours. What that means is that six hours after you have had a coffee, there is still 50 percent of the caffeine traveling through your body, keeping your body alert. And you still have 25% of it flowing through your body 12 hours later. If you are having trouble waking up feeling well rested, take a look at how you consume caffeine with this new knowledge. For instance, you most likely wouldn't drink half a coffee right before you go to bed. But if you drink a coffee at 4:00 PM, you still have half of that caffeine in your body at 10:00 PM. Which would essentially be like drinking half a cup of coffee and then trying to go to bed. I am sure not many of you would do that and expect to sleep well!

The topic of sleep has garnered a lot of interest and research, and we know a lot about how to achieve a good night's sleep. I wanted to give you a couple of places to start because it is so important for us. I am giving you a good place to start, as the topic of sleep is too big for me to cover all of it in this book. If you would like to dig deeper into this topic, please read Matthew Walker's book "While We Sleep". Working toward achieving a good night's sleep could be one of the most beneficial efforts you make.

Breathing

One of the most powerful tools we have for regulating our nervous system and managing our stress response is breathing.

Both the sympathetic and parasympathetic parts of our autonomic nervous system can be affected by how we breathe. When we breathe slowly and deeply, we turn on the parasympathetic nervous system. This helps to calm the body and make us feel more relaxed. This can help reduce stress and anxiety, as well as lower blood pressure and slow the heart rate.

On the other hand, when we breathe quickly and shallowly, we activate the sympathetic nervous system, which is associated with the "fight or flight" response. This can increase stress and anxiety, raise blood pressure, and accelerate the heart rate.

If we aren't breathing properly, we can have too much carbon dioxide in our bodies. When levels of carbon dioxide are too high, it can cause an increase in blood acidity, which can activate the sympathetic nervous system and increase feelings of stress and anxiety. This is why it's critical to breathe deeply and regularly to help eliminate excess carbon dioxide from the body and maintain a healthy oxygen-carbon dioxide balance.

Breathing can also have an impact on our mood. Deep breathing can aid in the release of endorphins, which are natural mood-enhancing chemicals in the brain. This can help lift our spirits and promote feelings of well-being.

Another important aspect of breathing is that it can help us focus and concentrate better. We can train our minds to be more focused and present in the moment by taking slow, deep breaths and focusing our attention on our breath.

I want to teach you two ways to breathe that have helped me and my clients significantly.

Physiological Sigh

The first technique I want to teach you is called the physiological sigh. This breath technique is the quickest and most reliable way to activate the parasympathetic nervous system (rest and digest), according to a recent study by Dr. Andrew Huberman and his lab. I can attest that it is a very effective technique, and I use it on a daily basis.

We will be breathing in through the nose and out through the mouth. We will complete one long inhale followed by another short inhale. This ensures we fill our lungs more than we would with a single, slow breath. We want to do this because when we are in a sympathetic state, the parts of the lungs that take in oxygen and release carbon dioxide can collapse and begin to work inefficiently. As the alveoli are critical to maintaining normal levels of oxygen and carbon dioxide in the body, it is important that they are functioning correctly.

The second inhale helps us to inflate our lungs more and helps to open up the alveoli. After our inhalation, we want to exhale slowly through the mouth. Our exhale should be at least two times longer than our inhale, but not too long, as we will start to feel out of breath. A 1-2 or 1-3 ratio of inhalation to exhalation is ideal. I mentioned early that our breathing patterns affect our nervous system. More specifically, when we breathe in, our chest expands and the pressure around the heart lowers.

To maintain blood pressure in the body, our hearts need to speed up, which in turn triggers a sympathetic response. When we breathe out, the pressure in our chests and our hearts increases, and the heart begins to slow down, triggering a parasympathetic response. So by having a 1-2 or even a 1-3 ratio, we are stimulating the parasympathetic system more than the sympathetic, resulting in a net positive effect of parasympathetic stimulation.

This technique can be used anytime you want! In Huberman's study, participants were asked to do 5 minutes of breathing a day with this technique. What they found was that not only did this breathing technique provide immediate relief, but the participants had overall lower levels of stress and slept better.

Box Breathing

The second most effective breathing technique in Huberman's study was box breathing. Box breathing is a technique where we breathe in for a specific amount of time, hold our breath for the same time, breathe out for the same time, and again hold our breath for the same period of time. This technique helps us in a number of ways. The deep and cyclical breathing helps us stimulate the parasympathetic nervous system and enter states of deeper relaxation. It also helps us with something called carbon dioxide tolerance.

Because carbon dioxide regulates the pH balance of the blood and brain tissue, having a high carbon dioxide tolerance is important for nervous system health. The nervous system, particularly the brain, is extremely sensitive to pH changes, and even minor variations can have a significant impact on brain function.

When CO_2 levels in the blood rise, the body responds by breathing faster to get rid of the extra CO_2 and keep the pH level stable. But if a person has a low carbon dioxide tolerance and feels uncomfortable or anxious when CO_2 levels rise, they may breathe more quickly, hyperventilate, and exhale too much CO_2, which can lead to hypocapnia (low carbon dioxide levels).

Hypocapnia can cause the narrowing of blood vessels in the brain, reducing blood flow and oxygen delivery and causing dizziness, confusion, and even loss of consciousness. Furthermore, hypocapnia can disrupt the balance of neurotransmitters in the brain, such as serotonin and GABA, aggravating symptoms of anxiety, depression, and other neurological disorders.

So, a high carbon dioxide tolerance can help keep the pH levels in the body and brain at a healthy level, which is important for the health of the nervous system and the body as a whole.

There is a test to see what your current level of carbon dioxide tolerance is. I want you to inhale and exhale deeply four times. After you have made your last inhalation, I want you to breathe out as slowly as possible and time it. The longer you can extend that exhalation, the better your tolerance.

There are a number of factors that can affect your tolerance, and stress and anxiety are two of the main ones. To give you some guidelines, if your exhalation was less than 40 seconds, we would consider this a low carbon dioxide tolerance. Forty to sixty seconds is fairly average, and anything over 80 seconds would be considered very good. You should do this test to determine how long your breaths should be in box breathing.

If you are in the lower category, your box breathing would take 2-3 seconds. Average 3-5 seconds, and if you are in the upper category, feel free to push yourself for longer breaths. You should choose a breath length that allows you to do box breathing for 5 minutes without feeling as if you are out of breath. So if you are in the middle category, you should breathe in for 5 seconds, hold for 5, breathe out for 5 and hold again. Keep repeating this pattern.

Heart Rate Variability

Heart rate variability (HRV) refers to the variation in the time interval between heartbeats. In other words, it is the change in the time between each heartbeat rather than the actual heart rate that is of interest. HRV is controlled by the autonomic nervous system (ANS), which regulates many of the body's internal functions, including heart rate, blood pressure, and breathing.

HRV is a useful way to figure out how well the sympathetic and parasympathetic parts of the ANS are working together. The sympathetic branch is responsible for the "fight or flight" response, while the parasympathetic branch is responsible for the "rest and digest" response. When the sympathetic and parasympathetic branches are in balance, HRV tends to be high. Conversely, when one branch is dominant over the other, HRV tends to be low.

HRV is important for the nervous system's ability to self-regulate because it shows how well the ANS can adapt to changes in the environment and keep body functions in balance. A high HRV indicates that the ANS is flexible and able to respond to stressors effectively, while a low HRV indicates that the ANS may be less adaptable and more susceptible to stress-related disorders.

Earlier in the book, I mentioned something called the vagal brake and that I was going to teach you an exercise to improve your vagal brake. HRV and the vagal brake are intimately connected because our HRV will reflect the interplay between our sympathetic and parasympathetic control of heart rate. The vagal brake is an important component of this interaction because it allows the parasympathetic branch to slow down heart rate during rest and recovery periods, thereby increasing HRV.

In healthy people, the vagal brake is a strong and flexible system that helps keep the sympathetic and parasympathetic parts of the autonomic nervous system (ANS) in balance. However, in people with autonomic dysfunction, the vagal brake may be impaired, resulting in a lower HRV and an increased risk of cardiovascular disease.

So when our HRV is high, our body is better able to regulate itself. There is an organization in the United States that has been investigating HRV for many years, and they have developed ways for us to improve it. They actually have a device that you can connect to your ear, and it will show you it to you in real time, and their software application will guide your breathing to increase it. You don't need the device, and the breathing technique is actually quite simple. The practice is made up of two parts. The first is breathing, and the second is a visualization practice.

For the breathing practice, I want you to follow five rules.

1. Your breathing should be what we call diaphragmatic breathing. This means we are engaging our diaphragm when we breathe. The easiest way to know if you are breathing with your diaphragm is to put one hand on your chest and the other just above your belly button, and observe which hand moves first when you start to inhale. If you are breathing with your diaphragm, your breath should start in the lower ribcage or belly and expand upwards to fill your chest. If the hand above

your belly button moves first, then the chances are good that you are using your diaphragm. If your chest moves first, then most likely you aren't breathing with your diaphragm. If you are a chest breather, you should practice breathing so that your belly and lower ribcage move first. Most of my clients found it easiest to practice this technique lying down.

2. Your breath should be taken in and out through the nose. If you have difficulty breathing through the nose, you can use your mouth; however, you will have better results breathing through the nose.

3. Your breath should be silent. If I was sitting beside you, I should not be able to hear your breath!

4. Your breath should be cyclical. You should not have any pauses between the inhalation and the exhalation, and vice versa. Over time, as you learn how to do this, your control over your diaphragm will greatly increase, and you will get even more benefit from this practice.

5. Your inhalation and exhalation should be the same length. The length of your breath should be as long as possible without you feeling out of breath. Some of my clients started with 2-second inhales and 2-second exhales and within a short period of time were able to reach 5-second inhales. It is more important to focus on the 5 rules, and over time, your breath will naturally get longer.

What the people at HeartMath also found was that, in addition to the breathing practice, if you are able to connect to feelings of joy, gratitude, love, etc., this produced a further increase in HRV. So what we want to do is find a quiet place and start to focus on our breath, following the five rules.

Once we start to feel more relaxed and our breath is flowing, I want you to visualize something (a person, a pet, a memory, an upcoming event, etc.) that you have a positive feeling towards. Keep breathing and focusing on this visualization. You may start to feel changes in your body and energy moving through your nervous system. I typically feel a warm feeling in my chest and a general relaxation throughout my body. If you don't feel any changes, don't worry. You will over time. A little trick I use sometimes is to put a big smile on my face. That usually produces a very nice feeling in my body!

Heat and Cold Exposure

Cold exposure has been one of the best ways for me to deal with stress and anxiety. In cold therapy, the body is exposed to cold temperatures, either by being submerged in cold water or by being exposed to cold air. The body's reaction to cold exposure can have profound effects on the nervous system, resulting in improved mood and resilience.

Cold therapy benefits the nervous system by causing the release of norepinephrine, a neurotransmitter that is important in mood and attention regulation. Norepinephrine is also involved in the body's stress response, and cold temperatures can help strengthen the body's ability to cope with stress.

Cold therapy also causes the body to make more endorphins, which are natural painkillers that can make you feel better and less anxious or sad.Endorphins have also been shown to improve resilience, or the ability to recover from stress and adversity.

Before you start cold therapy, you need to make sure you are safe by taking certain steps. If you don't have any underlying conditions, you can begin with brief exposure to cold temperatures, increasing the duration and intensity gradually over time. If you have any underlying health conditions, such as heart or circulatory issues, you should consult your doctor before beginning cold therapy. I would recommend finding a trained practitioner to help you determine if and how to start cold therapy.

Cold therapy can be very good for your nervous system and overall health. It can improve your mood, make you stronger, and rid you of the symptoms that accompany anxiety and depression.

Most of the time, heat therapy involves putting the body in a dry or wet sauna where the temperature is high. The body's reaction to heat exposure can have a significant impact on the nervous system, leading to improved mood and resilience.

Using a sauna is good for the nervous system because it makes the body release heat shock proteins, which are protective proteins that help fix damaged cells and improve the way they work. Heat shock proteins also have anti-inflammatory properties, which can aid in reducing inflammation and improving overall health.

Levels of endorphins, which are natural painkillers that make you feel good and reduce anxiety and depression, are also increased when you use a sauna. Endorphins have also been shown to improve resilience, or the ability to recover from stress and adversity.

Sauna use also benefits the nervous system by increasing heart rate and blood flow, which can improve cardiovascular health and lower the risk of heart disease.

It is critical to take certain precautions before beginning sauna use to ensure your safety. Begin with brief high-temperature exposure and gradually increase the duration and intensity over time. If you have any underlying health conditions, such as heart or circulatory issues, you should consult your doctor before beginning sauna use.

Rosenberg Exercise

Stanley Rosenberg is an author and craniosacral therapist who developed some techniques to improve the health of the vagus nerve. Earlier, I mentioned that the vagus nerve starts at the base of the brain and travels down through the neck before wandering throughout the abdomen. If we have a lot of tension in the neck, particularly at the base of the skull, it can negatively impact the vagus nerve.

Rosenberg developed a simple exercise to help release tension in the sub-occipital muscles located at the base of the skull. It also helps to release tension in the muscles of the eyes and the optic nerve. As we release the tension in these areas, we will elicit a response via the vagus nerve to engage the parasympathetic nervous system and, in turn, feel more relaxed. Don't let the simplicity of the exercise fool you. This is one of my favorites! Here is what you need to do:

1. You can do this exercise either while lying down or sitting.
2. Clasp your fingers together and place them at the base of your skull.
3. Take a few deep breaths and try to relax.
4. Look as far to the left as you can with only your eyes (without straining) and hold your eyes there for 30 to 60 seconds. You can do this with your eyes open or closed; however, I would recommend keeping them open. Make sure that your face is still pointed toward the ceiling.
5. Return your eyes to a neutral position and take a few deep breaths.
6. Look as far as you can with only your eyes (without straining) to the right and hold your eyes there for 30–60 seconds.
7. Return your eyes to a neutral position and take a few deep breaths.

Repeat as often as you need to until you feel the tension go away or your body starts to calm down. It's very common to yawn during this exercise, and this is a good sign you are moving into a parasympathetic response.

Diaphragmatic Breathing / Connection

In the first section on breathing techniques, I mentioned that we should be using our diaphragm to breathe. This may be a challenge for you for one of three reasons. The first is that your habitual way of breathing is more chest focused and you have never learned to breathe with your diaphragm.

The second is that the connection from your brain to the nerves that control the diaphragm is not developed enough for you to consciously use the muscle to control breathing. The third is that you may have a lot of tension in the rib cage and the diaphragm muscle, which makes it very difficult to use the diaphragm to breathe properly. In order to address issues of nervous system connection and control, you should practice the 5 rules of breathing listed in the first section on breathing. This method will help you consciously connect to the diaphragm and, over time, increase the connection and control of the diaphragm.

To address the issue of a tight or blocked diaphragm, there are a couple of simple exercises you can do to massage and release the diaphragm. Please be very gentle while doing these exercises.

1. Sit upright in a chair and begin to connect with your breathing. Once your breathing has slowed and you feel yourself beginning to relax, you can start the exercise. I want you to breathe in as deeply as possible. Filling your chest with as much air as possible. Then I want you to hold your breath and create pressure in your lungs and torso. We do this by keeping our mouth closed and trying to breathe out. Don't let any air escape from

your nose or mouth. At this point, you will want to start making a circular movement with your lower ribcage. Please start this exercise very gently, as if you exert too much effort, you may become quite dizzy and lightheaded.

2. After you have completed three to five repetitions of the first exercise, we are not going to use our hands to physically release the diaphragm. I want you to straighten your hands and make sure all of your fingers are together. Bend your fingers back towards your wrist so that they make a 90-degree angle with your palm. You are then going to gently place your fingers at the edge of your abdominal muscles and slightly beneath the ribs. Then you will lean forward, placing the backs of your hands on your thighs, and lean forward slightly so your fingers go a little deeper below your ribs. Stay in this position and breathe with your diaphragm. The tension of the diaphragm against your fingers will act as a gentle mass and stretch to help start unblocking your diaphragm. Please be very gentle here. If there is pain or it feels very uncomfortable, please try this with less pressure. If you can't find a level of pressure that feels good to you, then work with exercise number one for some time and then come back and try this exercise. This is a very vulnerable part of the body, and for many, it takes some time to build up the ability and confidence to do this exercise correctly. Please watch the video for a demonstration and more instructions.

Polyvagal Theory Mapping

As you begin to understand Polyvagal Theory and how your nervous system reacts to your world, you will start to notice that things fall into one of two categories. The first category is things that move you down the ladder (sympathetic response). The second category is things that move you up the ladder (parasympathetic response).

Deb Dana, in her book "Polyvagal Theory in Therapy" calls these "Triggers" and "Glimmers". I want you to start making a list of the things in your life that fall into these categories. The idea is that as you become aware of what things fall into either category, you can start making adjustments wherever possible in your life to remove the things that are triggering you and work to incorporate more of the things that move you up the ladder.

The idea is not to try to eliminate all of the triggers and make a perfect life with no problems. This would be great, but it is realistically not possible. Focus on the areas where you can make the changes, and you will find that over time, the program in your nervous system will start to be a more positive one. If you need more clarification, I would suggest rereading the chapter on Poly-Vagal Theory again for more information. It is a fairly straightforward and simple exercise that can have a profound impact on your life!

Music: Marconi Union

Music has a powerful effect on the vagus nerve, especially when it comes to promoting relaxation and stress reduction. You may already have some songs that you listen to to help you calm down.

Listening to slow, calming music has been shown in studies to help slow down our heart rate and breathing, which in turn can activate the vagus nerve and promote relaxation. This is commonly referred to as "music-induced relaxation."

There is also evidence that certain types of music, such as classical and meditation music, may be especially effective at stimulating the vagus nerve and promoting relaxation. As musical tastes are all different, what works for one person may or may not work for another. There is an abundance of music available to you to help create a relaxed feeling in the body.

I hope the song I am going to recommend helps you regulate your nervous system, but if it doesn't, please experiment a little to find a song that works for you. Listening to a calming song when you are stressed is a low-effort way to help regulate your body. I like to use relaxing music right before I go to bed (I combine it with the physiological sigh) to help regulate my nervous system and ensure I get the best sleep possible.

The song "Weightless" by the band Marconi Union is what I would like to recommend to you. This is a song that was specifically designed to elicit a parasympathetic response in your body and help you relax. The group that created "Weightless", did so in collaboration with sound therapists. The music is arranged so that it helps slow your heart rate, reduce blood pressure, and lower levels of the stress hormone cortisol. After the song was finished, a study was done to see if this song was effective in reducing the level of anxiety in the listeners. This study showed that participants felt a 65% reduction in anxiety after listening to this song.

I have used this song for years to help me relax when I need it. I have also recommended it to countless people, and they have also reported back to me that they noticed significant improvements in their anxiety as well. You can find the song on YouTube, Spotify, Apple Music, etc. I hope you enjoy it!

Humming / Chanting

Humming can stimulate the vagus nerve, which, as you now know, is one of the key components of the parasympathetic nervous system that regulates several vital bodily functions, including digestion, heart rate, and respiratory rate.

When we hum, the vibrations produced create a gentle, massage-like effect on the vocal cords and the muscles of the throat, which in turn activates the vagus nerve. When the vagus nerve is activated by humming, it can help our body relax and reduce feelings of stress and anxiety. This is because the vagus nerve can slow down our heart rate and lower our blood pressure, which makes us feel calmer and more relaxed.

If you look at the picture of the vagus nerve from Chapter 3, you can see that it is not only in our throat but also in our chest and abdomen. The humming exercise I am going to teach you will allow you to stimulate it in all three parts of the body. By gently massaging and stimulating the entire vagus nerve, we can increase the calming effect that humming produces.

There has actually been research on the effects of humming, and it has shown that regular humming can have several health benefits, including improving lung function, reducing stress and anxiety, and even enhancing memory and cognition.

For example, a study published in the International Journal of Behavioral Medicine in 2010 found that humming at a low pitch for just five minutes can increase heart rate variability (HRV), which is an indicator of vagus nerve activity. The study suggests that humming may be a simple and effective way to stimulate the vagus nerve and improve the body's ability to deal with stress.

In 2013, the International Journal of Neuroscience published the results of another study that found that humming can increase the amount of nitric oxide in the nasal passages. This is thought to stimulate the vagus nerve. This increase in nitric oxide may help reduce inflammation in the body and improve overall health.

Our exercise is going to have us humming the word AUM. We will first hum the "A" sound, followed by the "U" sound, and finally the "M" sound. Each of these sounds produces a vibration in a different part of the body. The "A" sound will create vibrations in the abdomen, the "U" sound in the chest, and finally the "M" sound will create vibrations in the throat. By combining all three, we can gently massage the entire vagus nerve and help us stimulate the rest and digest states in the body.

You can do this exercise sitting down or standing. Find a place where you won't be disturbed, and you can perform this exercise while standing, sitting, or laying down. Once you are comfortable, you will open your mouth and gently start humming the A-U-M sounds to create vibrations in the various parts of the body. So you would start with "aaaaaaa" then move to "uuuuuuu" and finally "mmmmmmm". Make sure you are producing the vibrations in the correct part of the body.

This may take some practice, but once you have figured out how to do it, this is a great exercise to help regulate your body. You can hum all three sounds within one breath, or you can do one sound, take a breath, and then move onto the next one. I would suggest that your session be at least 5 minutes; however, you may need more or less time until you start to feel the sense of relaxation start.

Gargling

Gargling can also stimulate the vagus nerve in a way very similar to humming because when we gargle, the muscles in our throat contract and relax, which creates vibrations that can activate the vagus nerve. The amount of time required for gargling to have an effect on the vagus nerve varies from person to person and is dependent on factors such as the substance used for gargling and the strength of the gargle.

According to research, gargling for as little as 30 seconds to 1 minute may be enough to activate the vagus nerve and produce beneficial effects on the body. For example, a 2013 study published in the International Journal of Medical Sciences discovered that gargling with salt water for 30 seconds can increase heart rate variability and activate the vagus nerve, which can aid in the reduction of inflammation and improve overall health.

Bonus Exercises
Muscle Relaxation Techniques

In the video course, I am including a set of bonus exercises that will help you release tension in your face, jaw, neck, and shoulders. Many of us carry a lot of tension in these areas, and over time, this tension can become habitual. We have spoken about how we program our nervous system to act in certain ways over time. These patterns extend to our muscles as well, and I am going to teach you a technique to release this tension so we can reprogram your nervous system so that this habitual tension goes away.

The technique is called pandiculation, and if you have animals at home, you will have seen them stretch this way. Pandiculation helps us improve the nervous system's control of the muscles. When you pandiculate, you engage both the voluntary and involuntary nervous systems, which aid in brain-muscle communication.

During the contraction phase of pandiculation, the nervous system sends a message to the muscle to contract. This contraction stimulates the sensory nerves within the muscle, which send information to the brain about the position and tension of the muscle.

During the release phase of pandiculation, the muscle slowly lets go. This turns on the involuntary nervous system. This system regulates the body's automatic, reflexive responses, including the stretch reflex. The stretch reflex is a protective mechanism that keeps muscles from becoming overstretched and injuring themselves. When a muscle is rapidly stretched, the reflex response is triggered, resulting in a quick contraction to protect the muscle. This involuntary system is what is responsible for the habitual tension that we have in the muscles, and by working with it, we can reprogram it to create less tension in the muscles.

Pandiculation helps the brain and muscles talk to each other better, which makes it easier to control and coordinate your movements. This can help reduce muscle tension and improve how well muscles work in general. Furthermore, regular pandiculation practice can help to retrain the nervous system to maintain optimal muscle length and tension, lowering the risk of injury and improving overall mobility.

Please view the videos for instructions and demonstrations of the various exercises.

You can also visit my website at www.wellnessiswithinyou.com to keep up to date with my work.

Access Your Exercise Demonstration and Instruction Video With This QR Code

Printed in Great Britain
by Amazon